DIET AND HEALTH

Alison Dalgleish

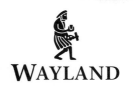

WAYLAND

Editor: Carron Brown
Designer: Rita Storey, StoreyBooks
Cover Designer: Giles Wheeler, Dome Design
Production Controller: Carol Titchener

The publishers would like to thank the staff and pupils of Uplands School in Brighton for their advice and support.

First published in 1997 by Wayland Publishers Ltd, 61 Western Road, Hove, East Sussex, BN3 1JD
Find Wayland on the internet at http://www.wayland.co.uk

British Library Cataloguing in Publication Data
Dalgleish, Alison
Diet and Health. – (Face the Facts)
   1. Diet – Juvenile literature 2. Health – Juvenile literature
   I. Title
   613'.0433
ISBN 0 7502 1755 3

Typeset by Storeybooks, England
Printed and bound by G. Canale in Turin, Italy

Picture acknowlegements

Danny Allmark *cover*, 12, 13, 17 (both), 19 (top), 22, 23, ; Sally and Richard Greenhill 9, 11, 20, 21, 25, 34 (bottom); Image Bank 36; Impact/Peter Arkell 32, /Nigel Davies 40; Life File/Juliet Highet 28, /David Kampfner 35, /Nigel Shuttleworth 27; Reflections Photo Library/Jennie Woodcock 38; Tony Stone/Christopher Bissell 5, 40 (top), /Ken Fisher 6, /Penny Tweedie 4, 26 (top), 31 (bottom), 39, /David Young Wolff 26 (bottom); Topham Picturepoint 14; Wayland Picture Library 7, 8, 15, 19 (bottom), 30, 31 (top), 34 (top), 43.
The illustrations on the title page and on pages 16, 18, 24, 29, 33, 37 and 42 are by Rachel Fuller.
Photo shoots directed by Bridget Tily.
Most of the people who appear in this book are models.
Thank you to the models and their agent Grace Jackman.

CONTENTS

BEING YOUR BEST
KNOWING YOURSELF

This book is about helping you to look your best and feel good about yourself. The ideas in this book will cover all aspects of you. Some you will feel happy with. Some you may want to know more about. Some you may want to change.

You can find a lot of information from books, but talking to someone at home or at school may help you more. That way your questions can be answered straight away.

▼ You are no longer a child but you are not yet an adult. Your body is changing, and so is the way you think about yourself and other people.

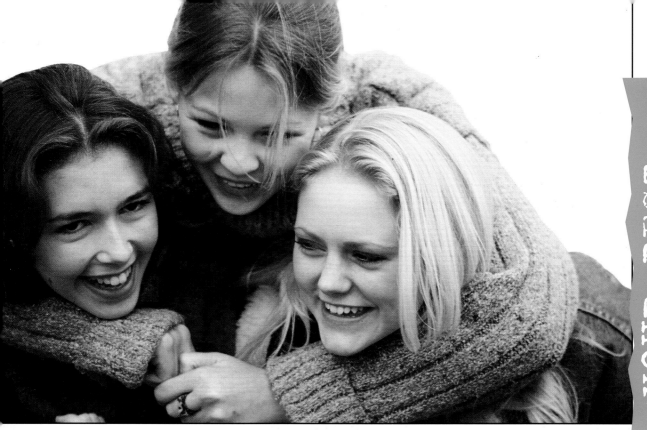

▲ Being with your friends, having fun and talking can make you feel happy.

How do I feel about myself and others?

DO I ALWAYS FEEL HAPPY?

YES! Great, that's a good start.

NO! Think. Is there a reason for this? Who can I ask to help me?

SOMETIMES! When do I feel content? Where do I feel relaxed? Who makes me happy? Why is this?

DO I ALWAYS FEEL HEALTHY?

YES! Great, you're a star!

NO! Perhaps I'm not eating properly, sleeping well, or having enough exercise.

SOMETIMES! When? After a long walk. If I don't eat chips too often. Where? On holiday or at school.

5

To be your best you need to find out the things that suit you. Everyone is different. You can have your own likes and dislikes in food, clothes, colours and interests.

If you want to change yourself, start by thinking about sensible changes that you can make. You can't, for example, change your height, your body frame or the colour of your skin. Think instead about the kind of person you are and what suits you.

How you feel about yourself is called your self-image.

How you look depends on your body, hair, face and clothes.

How you feel depends on your health, diet, sleep and exercise.

How you behave depends on your personality, interests, responsibilities and attitude.

Remember
even famous people dislike things about themselves. Sports people and film stars are paid to look good. So there's no point in trying to look that perfect.

66 Dawn: 'My life is changing in a lot of ways.' 99

Remember, if you spend your life comparing yourself to other people, it won't be surprising if you end up feeling miserable. Get to know yourself and what suits you. Then, as you begin to know what you want and like, you can feel more confident about yourself.

" John: 'I want to do things my way from now on.' "

Think about the things that suit you

- Talking.
- Following a leader.
- Being with other people.
- Things staying the same.
- Staying inside.
- Being quiet.

- Doing practical things.
- Taking the lead.
- Being on my own.
- A lot of changes.
- Being outdoors.
- A lot of noise and excitement.

LOOKING YOUR BEST
TAKING CARE OF YOUR BODY

Keeping clean

Personal cleanliness is very important. This means making sure that you keep your body clean.

Lack of personal hygiene can affect your health and the way you feel about yourself. It can also affect the way other people feel about you.

Having a bath or shower every day helps you feel fresh and clean. It makes you nice to be near.

If you can't have a bath or shower every day, try to have an all-over wash. It's important to make sure that your body is kept clean.

Hygiene

Hygiene is about being clean and staying healthy. In the teenage years, your body is starting to change because you are growing out of a child's shape into an adult's shape.

▼ It's great to have a bath or shower every day.

Body changes are brought about by new hormones in your body.

It will take some time for your body to adapt to the changes and for the newly working hormones to settle down.

Body changes

New sweat glands start working. They produce a heavier sweat.

The body often produces extra oil, called sebum. This makes the skin on the body and face more oily.

▲ Washing your face can remove extra oil.

Three reasons to take extra care over hygiene now

- To remove sweat and so stop body odour.
- To remove extra oil on the face and body.
- To remove dead skin cells on the body surface.

Basic body care

Keeping your body clean doesn't have to cost a lot.

- These are the basic items that you need: soap, sponge or flannel, deodorant, talc and nail brush.
- Luxury extras could be: bubble-bath or bath oil, shower gel, body spray, hand or body lotion.
- Items in fancy wrapping, or those which are perfumed, are likely to cost more. Plain supermarket brands are usually cheaper and just as good for everyday use.
- Special body sprays or aftershaves should be saved to be used on special occasions. Ask for your favourite one if you are asked what you'd like as a present.

Good habits

Having a good wash first thing in the morning and last thing at night.
Washing your hands before eating.
Washing your hands after going to the toilet.
Why? Washing removes dirt, grease, sweat and germs.

> **Carl:** 'Since my voice changed, I sweat a lot during PE. Afterwards, I have a shower at school to make sure I smell fresh. I put on some underarm deodorant.'

Your face and skin

The skin on your face may be dry, greasy or both. Skin types are usually the same in each family. Check the face-cleaning products used by your parents or older brothers and sisters. Chances are they will suit your skin type too.

Eating a lot of fruit and vegetables might not keep spots away, but if you eat a lot of junk food and don't have enough sleep or fresh air, then your skin will probably look bad.

Beware of staying out too long sunbathing. The sun's rays can dry out your skin and you risk getting burnt.

▶ Tan slowly, using plenty of the sun cream that suits your skin type.

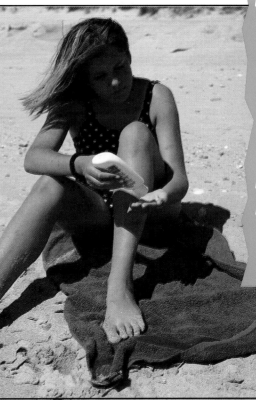

Skin types

Dry	Not enough oil. Sensitive to sun. Irritated by soap.
Oily	Too much oil. Shiny and greasy. Often gets spots and blackheads,
Part dry, part oily	The most common skin type. Greasy on forehead, nose and chin. Drier on cheeks.
Normal	Lucky you!

11

Boys' skin is thicker than girls' skin, and is usually firmer and stronger. It can still have the same spots though! Your skin can be protected by using moisturizer, and it's better to use unscented soap or cleanser to clean the face and neck.

The dreaded spots! Acne! Blackheads!

The truth is no matter how well it's looked after, your skin will normally cause you plenty of problems during your teens.

WHY?

Your body is producing a lot more hormones now. These stimulate your skin glands to produce more oil, called sebum. This is what encourages spots.

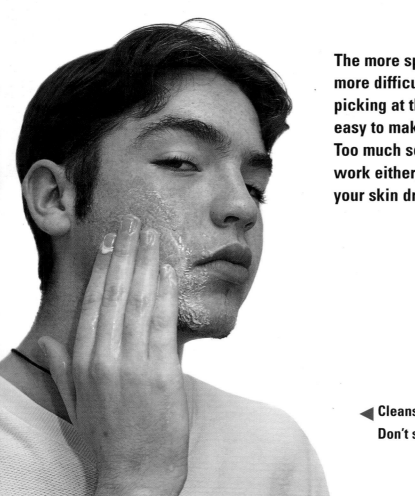

The more spots you get, the more difficult it is not to start picking at them. Then it's easy to make things worse. Too much scrubbing doesn't work either; it will only leave your skin dry and sore.

◀ Cleanse your face.
Don't scrub!

Some tips

- Make sure your hands and nails are clean. Gently squeeze out any blackheads then smooth antiseptic cream over the area.
- When a spot has a white head it can be gently squeezed. Never press hard until it bleeds.
- Check at the chemists for a good spot cream. Give it time to work.
- Get advice from your doctor about serious problems with spots and acne.

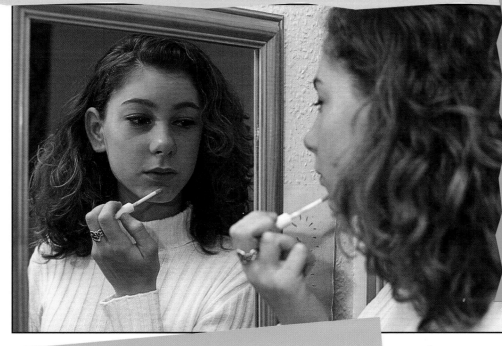

▲ Cover up spots for a while by using a special kind of make-up called concealer.

You're not alone!

Cheer up! Most teenagers have acne or spots at some time or another. Others know how it feels. It won't last forever. Between the ages of sixteen and twenty-five they will usually disappear.

Your mouth and teeth

Your mouth is one of the busiest parts of your body.

Good looks start with a great smile that shows healthy teeth.
Uncared-for teeth look nasty and can lead to bad breath.
There are no excuses for not having healthy teeth.
A check-up at the dentist and dental treatment is mostly FREE until
you are eighteen.

The dentist is there to help you to look after your teeth. So ask for help and advice when you go.

Plaque Food left on your teeth allows bacteria called plaque to coat your teeth. A build-up of plaque causes gum disease. It makes your gums bleed.

Decay Sugar in food and drink joins up with the bacteria in your mouth to make acid. This attacks the tooth enamel and burrows deeper to make holes in your teeth.

Tips for looking good when talking, laughing and kissing.

- Brush your teeth twice a day.
- Change your toothbrush every 6–8 weeks.
- Avoid sweets and fizzy drinks between meals.
- Try using dental floss to clean between your teeth.

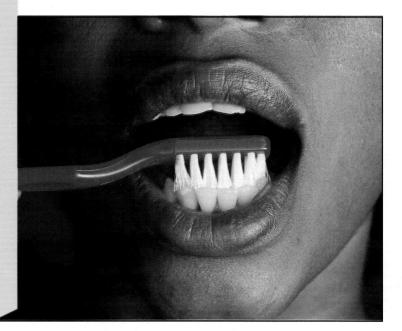

Eyes

Clear, bright eyes can make you look great.

The optician

Let your school or parents know straight away if you have a problem with your eyesight. It's best to go every two years to an optician. Having your eyesight tested is free while you are at school. An optician will test for: long sight, short sight, colour blindness and your ability to focus.

There are many different styles of glasses. You are sure to find a pair that really suits you. If you do have a problem wearing glasses, contact lenses may be the answer.

▼ About one in every five teenagers needs glasses.

The way to have great-looking eyes

- Having a good diet.
- Avoiding smoky places.
- Not watching TV or a computer screen for hours on end.
- Having the right amount of sleep.
- Not rubbing or touching your eyes too much.

Problem 'bits'

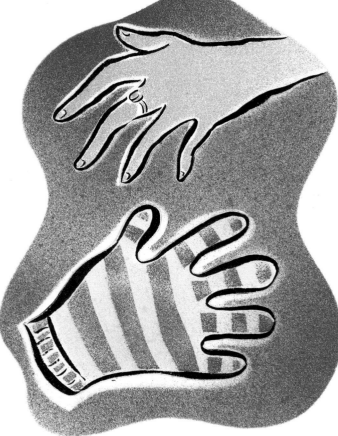

Hands

Hands need looking after sometimes. In the winter, they can become sore and the skin can become chapped. Wearing gloves when it's very cold can help. Also, try a hand cream or use Vaseline. Massage this into each hand. Keep nails short with nail trimmers or clippers.

Feet

Feet need a wash every day. There are a lot of sweat glands on the soles of your feet, and they can start to smell if not cleaned. Also, change your socks daily. Annoying problems, such as athlete's foot, verrucas, corns and blisters, can be avoided by good hygiene and wearing footwear that fits well.

Nails

Strong, glossy nails are a sign of good health. Strengthen them by eating more calcium. This is a mineral found in meat, milk, cheese, eggs and fish.

If you are a nail nibbler, it shows that you are a nervous person. Break the habit. Think of the dirt you're eating from under those nails. Find something else to do at times when you nibble the most.

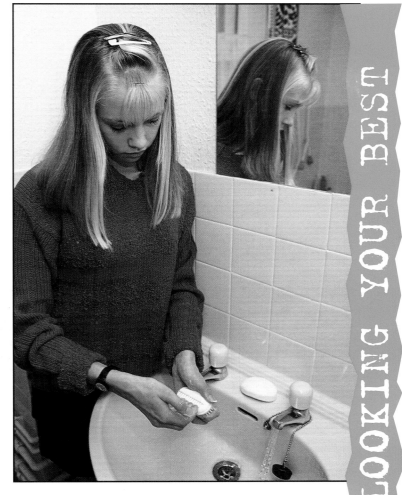

▲ Nails can be kept clean with a small nailbrush.

◀ Try painting your nails with a nasty-tasting, clear varnish.

17

WHAT TO WEAR?

Clothes

Wearing suitable clothes at certain times is important to keep yourself warm, dry or cool. The clothes you wear for school, for shopping or for a party will be different.

School clothes can wear out quickly because you wear them often.

Fashion or style

Fashion and style are not the same. What looks terrific on one person may look terrible on another. Wearing the latest fashion may not always suit your shape and colouring.

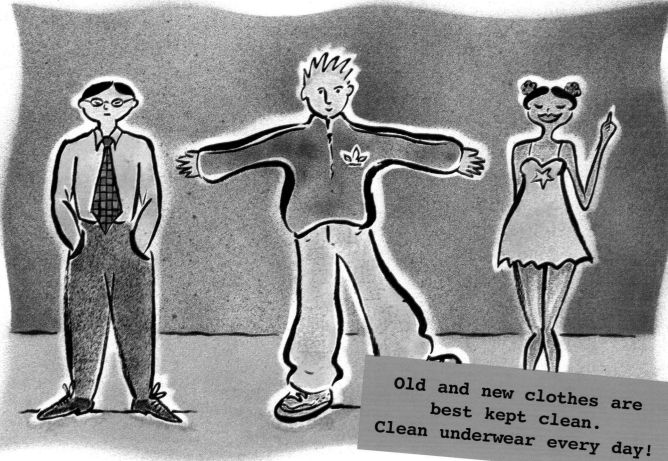

Old and new clothes are best kept clean. Clean underwear every day!

> **John:** 'I wear different clothes for different things. I like to wear jeans and a T-shirt on Saturdays when I go into town with my mates.'

> **Jenny:** 'I never wear my best clothes to school. I only wear my favourite top and smart trousers to school for the end of term party.'

Dressing well can be difficult for other reasons:

- If you're in a growing spurt, nothing fits for long.
- A lack of money holds you back from buying something you like.

Here are some decisions you can make:

- If someone is prepared to buy you some new clothes, ask to go with him or her. Don't wait to see what is brought home in the hope that you'll like it.
- Start finding out what suits you. Then, when you choose new clothes, you'll know what you want.
- When you go to buy clothes, spend time in the shop trying them on. Sizes can vary from shop to shop. It's best to go with a friend who can give you advice.
- Look at the clothes you already have. Buy clothes that match them and make up new outfits using your old clothes mixed with the new ones.
- Buy clothes and colours that make you feel happy, not fed up.

19

Basics

The basic clothes that form a wardrobe are simple tops, trousers and skirts. Never think of spending a lot of money on these clothes as they will be washed and worn often, and will need to be replaced eventually.

Extras

Extras, such as caps, hats, sunglasses, scarves and jewellery, can often be used to add to an outfit. Look for these on market stalls or in the sales.

Jeans last a long time. They can look good with smart tops or T-shirts. Even when jeans seem worn out, don't throw them away. Cut off the bottom part and see if they can be worn as shorts.

Bargains beware!

Look in your wardrobe before you go to the sales. Make sure you really need the item that you are tempted to buy. Check it for faults. Many items are cheaper because they are faulty.

Still try on before buying. Check if the item can be machine-washed. Think about the money you are spending, not how much you are saving. Most importantly, don't go to the sales if you're broke!

▶ It is easier to take care of clothes that can be machine-washed.

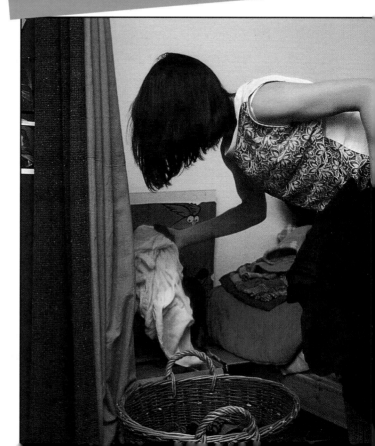

Footwear

Girls have more styles of footwear to choose from than boys. But your choice needs to be sensible and realistic for school. Go for brown or black if you can only afford one pair. Those colours will go with most clothes.

Leather shoes cost more, but are kind on the feet and last longer. They let feet 'breathe' and stop them from sweating a lot.

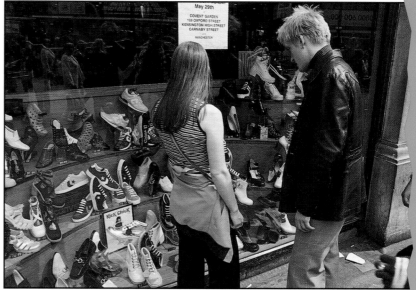

▲ Try on shoes before buying them.

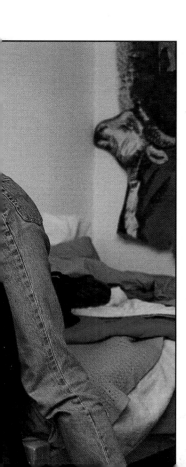

Trainers are popular. They are made to let your feet breathe too. But wearing them day in and day out will make your feet hot and sweaty.

Don't go shopping for shoes after doing a lot of walking. Your feet will be slightly bigger then.

Taking care of your clothes

Hang up your clothes when you take them off. If clothes are dropped on the floor, they will pick up dirt and crease quickly.

Outer clothes and shoes need to be aired at night. Clothes that touch your skin pick up some of your body dirt, sweat and dead skin cells. So underwear, shirts, socks and tights need changing every day.

HAIR CARE

Whether your hair is long, short, curly or styled, here's how to keep it looking good and feeling great.

Every day

Brush and comb well in the morning. Add a little gel, mousse or hairspray to keep it in place. For school, longer hair is probably easier to manage if you tie it back.

Every few days

Shampoo your hair to keep it clean and wash away all the spray and gel you've used.

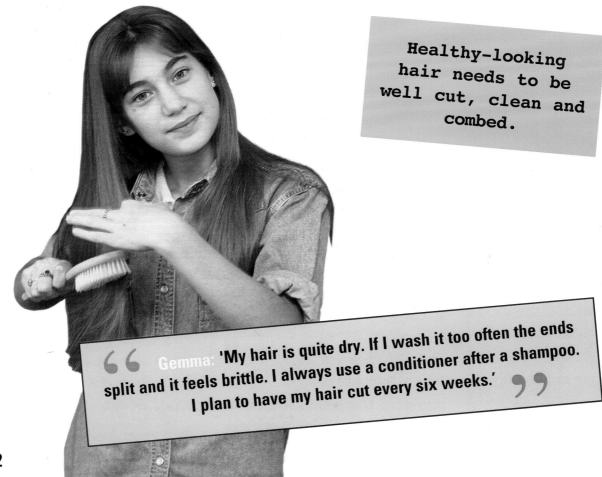

Healthy-looking hair needs to be well cut, clean and combed.

Gemma: 'My hair is quite dry. If I wash it too often the ends split and it feels brittle. I always use a conditioner after a shampoo. I plan to have my hair cut every six weeks.'

> 66 **Brett:** 'Keeping my hair stylish means a lot to me. I like to look smart. My hair is curly and I wash it every two days.
> I comb in some gel to get the right style.' 99

The clean hair guide

To clean your hair really well:

- Check first that it's really wet through before shampooing.
- Lather up well by massaging all over your scalp with the tips of your fingers.
- Rinse thoroughly. Check the water is running clear before you stop.
- If your hair is squeaky clean, there is no need to shampoo it again.

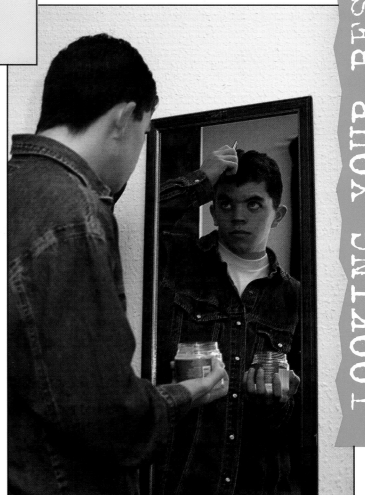

The cost

Supermarkets sell many hair-care products. Look out for dandruff shampoo and all-in-one shampoo and conditioner. It makes sense when you try out new shampoo to buy a trial size or a small size first. Consider buying shops' 'own' brands as they are usually good value for money.

The happy hair guide

For dry, brittle or frizzy hair add some conditioner after washing. Rub a small blob of conditioner over the palms of your hands and smooth it through your hair. Wait until it has soaked in, then rinse your hair again.

Hair can become damaged if you blow-dry it often. The only way to cure split ends is to have them cut off. A good trim every six weeks or so will do this.

Trying out new hair-styles at home using gloopy gel, sculpting lotion, wax or hold-fast hairspray can be fun.

Check with friends or family for a good hairdresser or barber to give you the haircut you want. Remember, some fashions and styles won't go down well at school.

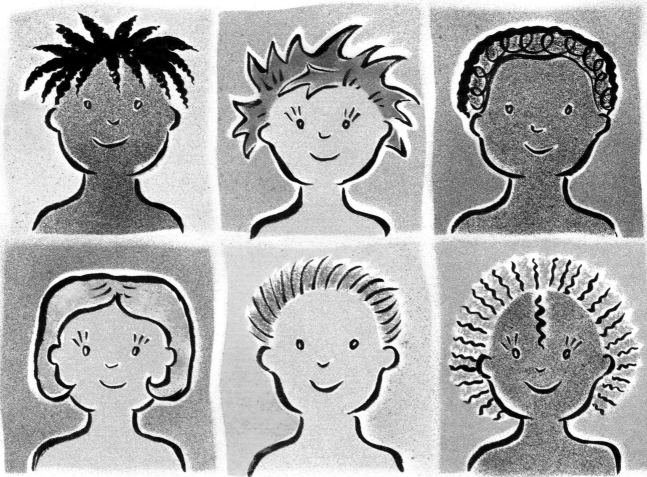

Hair helpline

'When I brush my hair, a lot seems to come out. Is this normal?'
You lose about a hundred hairs each day to make way for new hair. Brushing too hard or when hair is wet can pull out hair. So go gently.

'Help! I have dandruff.'
Try a gentle, frequent-wash shampoo. Massage your scalp as you wash your hair. Try a medicated or anti-dandruff shampoo for a while.

'I want a perm to make my hair curly, but it's so fine I'm scared it will go frizzy!'
A good hairdresser will be used to dealing with all hair types and perms to match. Check with friends who have the same hair type to see what they've tried.

'My hair is so curly. It drives me mad!'
Many hairdressers can do hair-relaxing styles. This can be costly though. Keeping your hair short and styling it each day can help.

'I want to colour my hair but my mum won't let me!'
It may be easier to talk your mum into letting you try a temporary hair dye. This will go after a few washes.

BODY DECORATION

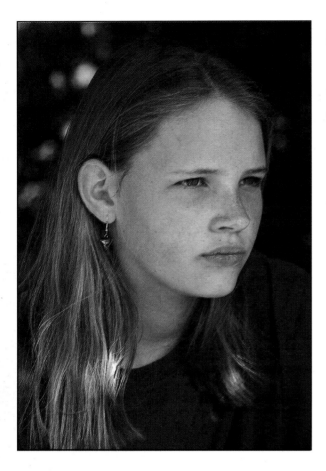

Ear piercing

Choosing to have your ears pierced in your teens, especially for boys, can be frowned upon by parents and schools. Check if this is the case and find out people's reasons for not liking ear piercing. You may decide to wait until you're a bit older.

◄ Go to an ear-piercing centre where everything used is clean to prevent infection.

◄ It is wise to check with parents and school before having your ears pierced.

Where to go to get your ears pierced

You risk getting an infection if you try to pierce your own ear. Instead, go to an ear-piercing centre. Many hairdressing salons have them. An ear-piercing gun, which fires a sterilized stud through your ear lobe, is used. Then you will have to be careful to keep your ears and earrings clean for at least six weeks.

Body piercing

Body piercing, such as nose piercing, carries the same risk of infection as ear piercing. Again, think carefully before having anything pierced. Check that your school and parents will allow you first, and then have it done at a special body-piercing centre where everything will be sterilized.

Tattoos

Tattoos are a very serious form of body decoration. They can't be washed off. It is also illegal to have a tattoo done before you are eighteen. If you know a place that will do it before this age, beware!

Risks

The most serious risk is of getting Hepatitis B or HIV from a needle that is not properly sterilized.

▶ A tattoo stays on your body for ever. It can't be washed off.

FEELING YOUR BEST
HEALTHY EATING

The food you like best may not always be good for you. Your body needs the right kind of food in the teenage years.

Why?
- To give you energy.
- To make you feel well.
- To keep your skin clear.
- To help you grow properly.

A healthy diet

This means eating the right kinds of food that your body needs while you are growing, such as fruit; fresh vegetables, eaten raw, lightly boiled or microwaved; bread and cereals, especially wholegrain; white meat, such as pork and skinless chicken; and fresh fish (not deep fried in batter).

If you can choose what to eat, try
- branflakes instead of bacon
- a banana instead of crisps
- salad instead of sausages
- jacket potato instead of chips

Why we need to eat

Everyone has to eat in order to live. You soon know when you feel hungry, but you have to decide the right kinds of food to eat to keep your body healthy. The purpose of food is to provide your body with some essential materials called nutrients.

◀ Eat an apple instead of sweets.

Nutrients are things that do a particular job in the body. To stay healthy we need a variety of these. Here are the most important ones:

TYPE	SOME FOODS IT IS FOUND IN	WHAT IT DOES
Protein	Nuts, fish, meat, eggs, dairy products, pulses, vegetables	Builds up and repairs the body. Provides energy.
Carbohydrates	Rice, pasta, potatoes,	Provides energy.
Fibre or roughage	Branflakes, bananas, wholemeal bread	Helps the body get rid of waste.
Fats	Dairy products, meat, nuts	Provides warmth and energy.
Vitamins and minerals	Liver, vegetables, fruit, milk	Protects against illness. Helps body to use other nutrients.

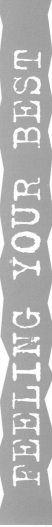

FEELING YOUR BEST

Drinks

Drinking plenty of water is good for your body. Coffee and tea contain a drug called caffeine that can give you energy for a while, then leave you feeling tired. Herbal tea or fruit juice is better for you.

Quality eating

Think about what you eat every day. Are you used to eating convenience or junk food? These are foods which are quick and easy to cook and eat but have few nutrients in them.

Are you eating a lot of chocolate, biscuits, cakes, tinned meats, packet soups, crisps and chips? These are foods that contain a lot of sugar, salt and fat, and are bad for you.

SUGAR warning!

- Sugar rots teeth!

- Sugar is very fattening!

- Sugar provides energy, but no other nutrients!

- Sugar can cause spots!

SALT warning!

- Too much salt leads to high blood pressure, which can cause health problems when you are older.

- It's easy to eat too much salt. Lots of snack food such as crisps are salty.

- Adding extra salt to a meal can spoil the real flavour of the food.

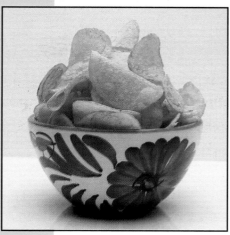

▲ Crisps contain salt. It's best not to eat too many salty snacks a day.

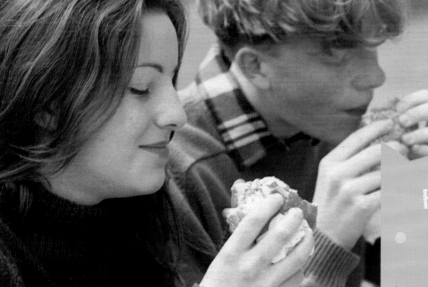

▲ Good or bad eating habits start when you are young.

Start noticing how often you eat high-fat foods, sweet, sugary foods and salty foods. Think about changing the balance if you eat more of these than healthy foods.

FAT warning!

- Fatty food contains cholesterol. This can cause heart disease.

- Eating a lot of fatty foods can make you overweight.

- Being overweight can cause heart disease.

Healthy eating from breakfast to bedtime

`Breakfast` Don't miss this meal because you're in a rush. You'll soon get hungry and start eating crisps and sweets at breaktime. Breakfast cereals are good for you and are quick and easy to eat. Many contain fibre, which helps your body to digest food.

`Packed lunch` If you make a sandwich, cut down on fat. Try using a low-fat spread. Some moist fillings, such as peanut butter and tuna, don't need butter added as well.

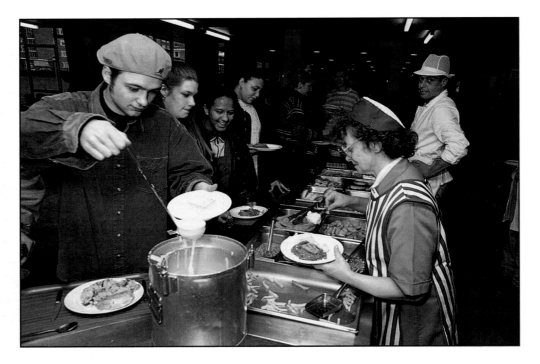

▲ Spend your money wisely. If you have a choice, don't always go for chips and fast-food. Most schools offer a healthier range of food.

`Snacks` Try fruit, nuts and raisins, or raw carrots sometimes. Break the habit of snacking on crisps, chocolate and fizzy drinks, and drink plenty of water. It's good for you as well as filling you up.

`Evening meal` Try to eat at least two hours before you go to bed. Give yourself a chance to burn off some of the calories.

Calories

The energy provided by food is measured in calories. Some foods, such as cheese, potatoes and chocolate, have a lot of calories. Fruit and most vegetables have only a few calories. As a teenager, you need plenty of high-calorie food to give you energy, but make sure you get your calories from healthy foods and exercise regularly. Eating foods with a lot of calories and not exercising can cause weight problems.

Crash diets

Eating a sensible diet and taking exercise should keep your weight at the proper level for your age. Dieting is not a good idea while you are still growing. As you grow taller you will find you become slimmer naturally.

A good diet will cut down on sugar and fats.

Cutting down on food altogether is a bad way to diet. Suddenly starving your body of food can be dangerous for your health.

If you think you are overweight for your height and build, or are worried about your weight at all, make an appointment with your doctor to talk about it.

EXERCISE AND REST

EXERCISE, whether it's a long walk or a game of football, is a great way of keeping healthy and helping your body feel good which also helps you to feel happy.

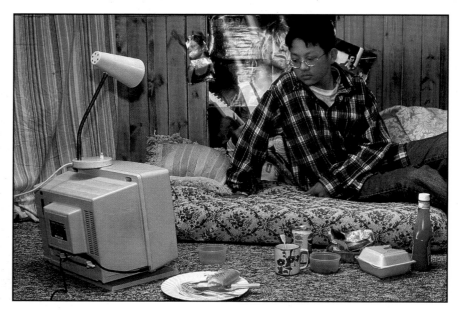

▲ If you are feeling down, doing exercise can lift your mood much better than sitting slumped in front of the TV.

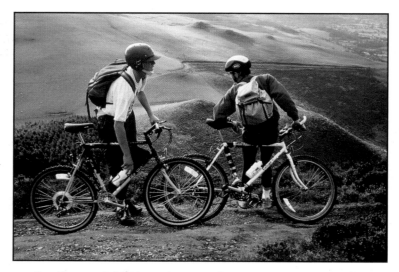

▲ Outdoor activities, such as cycling, provide exercise and fresh air.

Why bother to keep fit and healthy?

Being healthy means your body is in good working order. Fitness is how much you can do with your body. Fitness training can help you to do more and make you stronger and more supple. Being fit and healthy can help to improve the way you look. Your body firms up, and the condition of your skin and hair improves.

Exercise and body shape

Many teenagers would like to change their body shapes but do not like sport. But there are many different types of exercise, most of which are fun to do. Try hill climbing, ice-skating, roller-blading or swimming with a group of friends. There are also evening classes that teach yoga, judo and aerobics.

Think about cycling or walking to the shops, library or a friend's house. Always ensure you take a safe route or walk with someone. If you like to exercise alone, borrow an exercise tape or video and practise in your room.

Posture

Exercise starts with good posture. This is the way you hold yourself when you stand, sit and move. It can affect your digestion and feelings of energy and tension. Good posture can help to prevent backache. Exercise such as yoga, swimming, walking and stretching all strengthen your back and improve your posture.

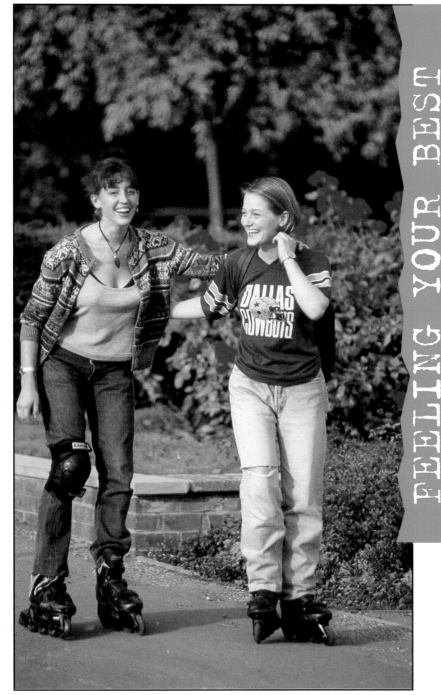

▲ Try roller-blading with your friends.

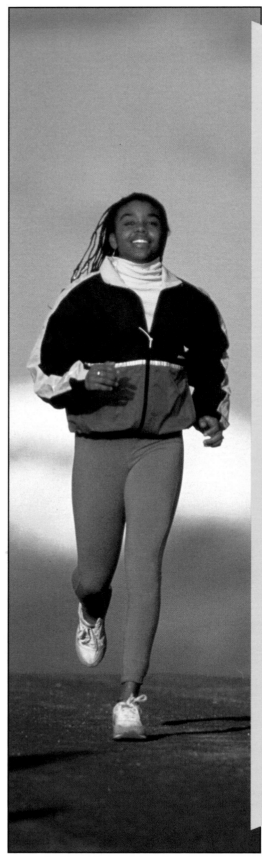

Regular exercise helps your body in three ways. It helps to give you stamina, strength and suppleness.

Stamina

If you have a lot of stamina, you can exercise for a long time without getting tired out. Aerobic activities improve stamina. These are exercises that make your heart pump and fill your lungs with plenty of air.
Exercise that helps to build up stamina: walking, jogging, skipping, swimming, cycling and aerobics.

Strength

Strength is the amount of force your muscles can produce. Without exercise, muscles become weak and flabby. There are over 600 muscles in the body that help you to move and breathe.
To develop muscles you need to make them work hard for a short period of time by doing exercise such as: swimming, weight-lifting, gymnastics, canoeing, rowing.

Suppleness

This is being able to bend and stretch easily. Trained dancers and gymnasts are very supple. Suppleness helps to prevent sprains and damage to your body.
Ways to become supple: gentle bending and stretching exercises, yoga, volleyball, skating, judo, tennis, all kinds of dancing and gymnastics.

▲ Jogging is an exercise that helps to build up stamina.

Rest and sleep

Having enough rest and sleep is important to stay healthy. As a teenager, you may find you need a lot of sleep because while your body is growing, you feel tired. Try to have seven to eight hours' sleep every night. If you've been out until late or studying late into the night, it will show the next day.

`Sleep` gives your body a chance to rest. Skin can renew itself. Your heart rate slows down. Muscles relax. You breathe slower and deeper.

If you find it difficult to sleep sometimes
- Try reading a book or magazine to calm your mind.
- Have a warm bath to help you relax.
- Have a hot, milky drink before going to bed.
- Take some exercise in the evening to help muscles relax. Try yoga or relaxation exercises.
- Avoid tea, coffee and food before bedtime.

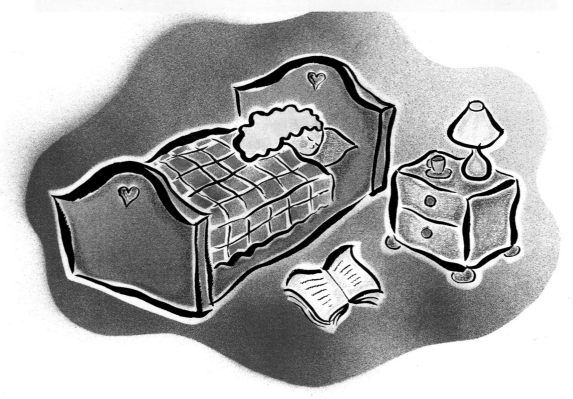

MAKING CHOICES ABOUT YOUR HEALTH

Drugs

If drugs are so bad for you, then why do so many people take them? Many people smoke cigarettes, which contain the drug nicotine, and drink alcohol. Some people take other drugs such as cannabis, Ecstasy and amphetamines, which are illegal. These are some reasons people take drugs: for excitement, a good feeling, for pleasure, to keep calm and in control.

> 66 **Darren:**
> 'It's my mind and body. Who says I can't? I'll try what I want! What else is there to do?' 99

Risks and dangers

There are many risks and dangers involved with drugs. You need to be aware of them to help yourself and other people. Legal drugs, such as cigarettes and

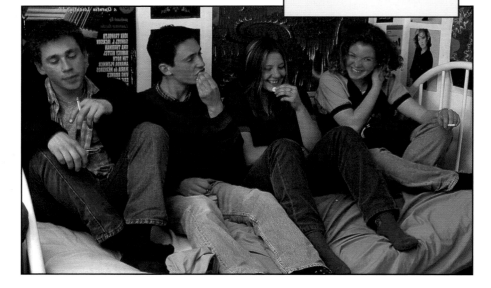

alcohol, may seem safe but are not. Nicotine in cigarettes can be highly addictive, and is harmful to smokers' health and those around them, causing illnesses like lung cancer. It's illegal to smoke until you are sixteen. Drinking alcohol can make you feel relaxed and happy. Drinking a lot very quickly can have the opposite effect. It can make you slur your words, lose your balance, be sick or pass out. You might do and say things you normally wouldn't. Sensible drinking is enjoyable. Have a glass of milk and eat something before drinking. It's best to drink at your own pace. It's illegal to drink alcohol until you are eighteen.

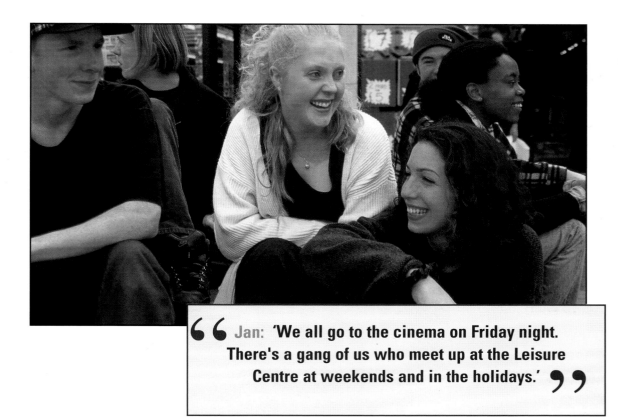

> 66 Jan: 'We all go to the cinema on Friday night. There's a gang of us who meet up at the Leisure Centre at weekends and in the holidays.' 99

`Illegal` `drugs` are dangerous because you don't know what is in them or how your body will react to them. If found taking them, you could be in a lot of trouble. Even medicines from the doctor or chemist can be dangerous if you don't follow the instructions. Always seek advice when offered drugs. Never be pushed into taking them, even if all your friends all do. Remember that every time you take a drug, you take a risk.

Safe choices

Drinking alcohol, taking illegal drugs, inhaling substances and smoking are some of the things you may have thought about trying. Exploring your body and experimenting with new and different things are part of growing up, and they may seem more exciting if adults disapprove. Yet always find out the dangers first and think carefully about what you are doing.

SHOWING YOUR BEST
YOUR CHANGING FEELINGS

The teenage years can be difficult because you are developing both physically and emotionally. Maybe you are a bit unsure of what is happening to you. You may feel unsure of yourself.

As you come to the end of this book, you should have some good ideas about how you can feel happy about the way you look. That is the first step to feeling confident about yourself both in and out of school.

Feeling confident

In safe and familiar places, such as home, you feel comfortable. Going out and facing new situations and people can be difficult.

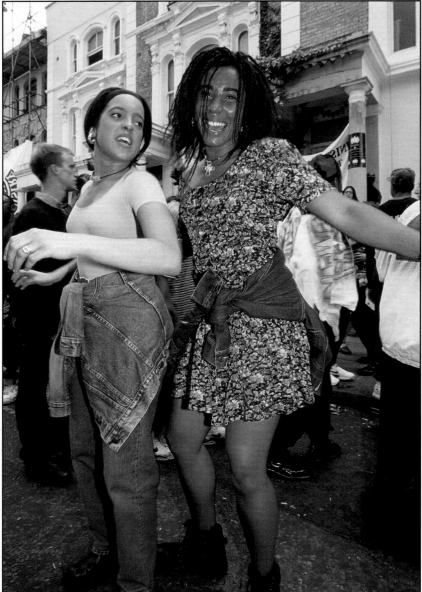

▲ Being happy about the way you look is the first step to feeling confident about yourself.

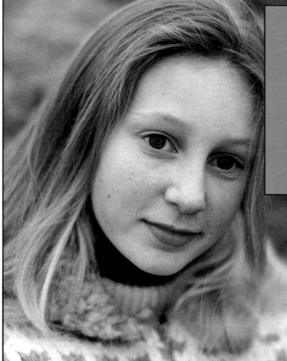

> 66 **Joanne:**
> 'I always blush when I have to speak. I can hear my heart beating like thunder and I start to stammer. Most of the time I don't say anything in case I make a fool out of myself. ' 99

What to do

Be positive about yourself. If you think that no one will want to talk to you, that you look bad, that you are going to have a terrible time, then more than likely you will.

Think of the good points, both of your looks and your personality. Everyone has good points. Stop feeling sorry for yourself and find a reason to feel good.

Remember everyone feels shy or worried about some things. Put on a bit of an act, and appear calm and confident. Start by smiling!

> 66 **Wayne:**
> 'I was on work experience and my hands went all clammy when I met the boss. I know it sounds silly, but I couldn't stop fiddling with my glasses.' 99

41

Body language

This is the signal you give by the way you look and hold yourself, and your movements or gestures. Even when you feel shy, your body language can show the opposite. This can help you through some sticky moments, such as talking in front of a group or joining a new club.

Positive signs
Smiling
Hands relaxed and lightly clasped
Uncrossed knees when sitting
Standing upright
Facing the person you're speaking to

Negative signs
Frowning
Avoiding eye contact
Crossing arms and legs tightly
Holding your hands in front of your
    face and mouth
Hunching your shoulders
Standing side on to the person
    you're speaking to
Fiddling with fingers, rings,
    clothing etc.

Emotions

Feeling strongly about issues, and rebelling against parents and other adults, have always been a part of teenage years. Use this energy in useful ways. Don't let it spoil your life. Keep busy and happy with some of the ideas in this book to help you.

Keeping safe

Rushing out of the house in a temper after an argument can put you in danger. It's better to go somewhere quiet, like your room, and let yourself calm down. Listen to some music perhaps. When you go out, always let someone know where you are, especially in the evenings. Have an emergency plan ready if things go wrong. It's far safer to phone home if you've missed the last bus, rather than accept a lift from a stranger. There are dangers in our society and you need to be aware of them.

Joining in with activities at school, and learning to get along with others by accepting that they have different ideas and opinions, form a valuable part of growing up. Knowing too that you can be fit and healthy can build up your confidence as you develop through the teenage years.

NOTES FOR PARENTS AND TEACHERS

KNOWING YOURSELF

This chapter is an introduction to physical and emotional changes. The questions on page five are to encourage pupils to discuss the differences in their thoughts and feelings now that they have reached puberty. Looking at photographs of themselves as young children and as they are now could be a visual starting point, leading to a comparison of their appearance and thoughts on school, home, food, exercise, behaviour, etc. The points on page seven, 'Think about the things that suit you', indicate that individual differences are natural. Ideas about self-image need explanation and discussion. In this chapter, the reader should discover that being liked and having self-confidence are linked with a whole range of things.

LOOKING YOUR BEST

TAKING CARE OF YOUR BODY

The main issue is one of greater need for personal hygiene because of body changes. It may be necessary to deal with boys' and girls' issues separately. Two excellent books written in very up-to-date, zappy style are *Style-Blitz – Grooming and Good Looks for Boys* by Helen Thorne and *Everything a Girl Should Know* by Samantha Rugen (see Further information, page 47). Other areas to discuss and expand on concern both sexes, i.e. skin care, teeth, eyesight, hands, feet, nails, ear and body piercing and tattoos.

WHAT TO WEAR

Most pupils probably won't have much freedom of choice, so taking care of their present wardrobes, discussion of appropriate clothes and footwear for different weather and occasions are the main issues. Extend this topic with discussion of body shape, 'puppy fat', size and how to measure the body so that clothes are bought in the right size.

HAIR CARE

There is likely to be a wide range of hair types in any group of people. Discussing the latest fashion and its merits could prove interesting. Emphasis here is on cleanliness and daily routine. The problem of head lice might need to be raised.

FEELING YOUR BEST

HEALTHY EATING

Ideas on achieving a balanced diet are the main concern. The chapter introduces basic nutritional information. The intention is to help readers to think about what they eat and the effect on their bodies. Preparing a blank weekly diet sheet for them to fill in could be a starting point. Readers could look at the nutrients in their week's food and discuss ways of improving their diets if necessary. The *Food Facts* pack, published by Cambridge Resource Packs, contains up-to-date information for parents and teachers. Extend the above information by looking at food labels to approach ideas on food additives and vegetarianism. Giving more information on the dangers of dieting is essential. *Dealing with Eating Disorders* by Kate Haycock and *We're Talking About Eating Disorders* by Rhoda Nottridge, both published by Wayland, provide useful information on eating disorders.

EXERCISE AND REST

A brief outline of the benefits of exercise is given. More details about the human body and the way it works could be given, plus practical activities to help explain stamina, strength and suppleness. Readers could list a range of sports and leisure activities available in the area using leaflets and information from the library. Further investigation could include sports programmes and videos to see different exercises in practice. The issue of athletes and body builders using performance-enhancing drugs could be raised.

MAKING CHOICES ABOUT YOUR HEALTH

The more information young people can be given about drugs the better. Research has shown that education about drugs is more effective in preventing misuse than saying 'don't do it'. Most teenagers will give drugs a try. Useful information is given in *Drugs Use and Misuse* published by The Chalkface Project and *Face the Facts: Drugs* published by Wayland. Giving information about AIDs and HIV is important. Advice, information and direct discussion with doctors needs to be offered.

SHOWING YOUR BEST

YOUR CHANGING FEELINGS

The final chapter explores ideas of coping with difficult situations where teenagers may feel shy, embarrassed and awkward. The readers should discuss one situation and how they felt. Start by identifying with the case studies. Depending on the group, it could be useful for readers to list their good and bad points, and practise body language in role-play situations. Discussing how to listen as well as talk, the range of emotions from anger to calmness, why some people annoy and others please and the reasons for this, could be useful for self-awareness. The idea that growing up and being more independent brings with it many responsibilities, and even dangers need to be explored in detail.

GLOSSARY

Anorexia nervosa

A condition where someone deliberately starves their body of food in order to control their weight. Sufferers of this serious eating disorder think they are fat when they are usually they are too thin.

Acne

A condition that causes spots in teenagers, especially on the face, neck, back and chest.

Athlete's foot

A condition that affects the feet, making the skin between the toes sore and flaky.

Attitude

Behaviour that reflects your opinions.

Blackheads

Pores in the skin that have been blocked up with dark sebum (oil).

Body frame

The shape of your body, made up of the structure of your bones, muscles and skin.

Bulimia

An illness that involves a person overeating then being sick to get rid of the food so that he or she doesn't gain weight.

Calories

The units in which the energy provided by food is measured.

Cholesterol

The substance in animal fats that can contribute to heart disease.

Diet

The foods that you eat regularly make up your diet.

Emotions

Strong feelings.

Hepatitus B

A disease that is passed on through blood often through infected needles.

HIV

Human Immunodefiency Virus. This virus, passed through body fluids such as blood, is the cause of AIDS.

Hormones

Chemical substances in the body.

Hygiene

Cleanliness.

Illegal

Something that is against the law.

Junk food

Food that is processed so that it is easy to prepare and cook, but contains very few nutrients.

Legal

Something that is allowed by law.

Nutrients

The elements of food that have a particular useful function in the body.

Posture

The way the body is positioned when standing, sitting and moving.

Stamina

The ability to continue exercising for a long time without becoming very tired.

Strength

Muscular power.

Suppleness

The ability to bend the body freely without damaging the joints.

Tooth enamel

The hard, glossy coating on the outside of a tooth that helps protect it from decay.

Verruca

A hard, contagious wart that affects the sole of the foot.

FURTHER INFORMATION

Books to read

Core Skills by T. & M. Ralph (Stanley Thornes, 1991)

Dealing With Eating Disorders by Kate Haycock
(Wayland, 1994)

Drugs Use and Abuse by Mike Dooling (The Chalkface Project, 1993)

Everything a Girl Should Know by Samantha Rugen (Piccadilly
Press, 1994)

Face the Facts: Drugs by Adrian King (Wayland, 1997)

Food Facts by Dr Gerald Beales (Cambridge Resource Packs, 1990)

Style Blitz – Grooming and Good Looks for Boys by
Helen Thorne (Piccadilly Press, 1994)

Vitamins by Rhoda Nottridge (Wayland, 1992)

We're Talking About Eating Disorders by Rhoda Nottidge
(Wayland, 1997)

Useful information

Health Education Authority
Hamilton House
Mabledon Place
London
WC1H 9TX
Tel: 0171 383 3833

National Centre for Eating Disorders
54 New Road
Esher
Surrey
KT10 9NU
Tel: 01372 469 493

Action on Smoking and Health (ASH)
5–11 Mortimer Street
London
W1N 7RH
Tel: 0171 637 9843

INDEX